SHOULDER PAIN

SHOULDER PAIN
TREATMENT GUIDE

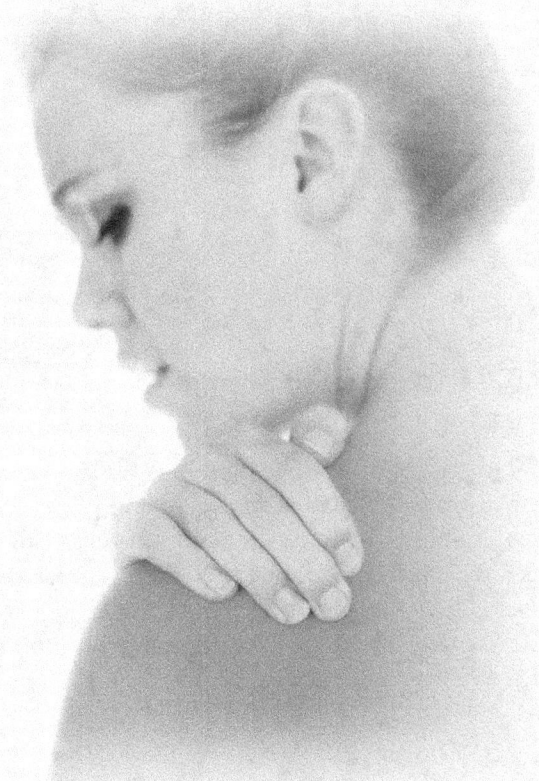

Get Relief Without Medications,
Injections, or Surgery

CHRIS DUKARSKI, PT

DISCLAIMER:

The information provided in this book is designed to provide helpful information on the subjects discussed. This book is not meant to be used, nor should it be used, to diagnose or treat any medical condition. For diagnosis or treatment of any medical problem, consult your own physician. The publisher and author are not responsible for any specific medical or health needs that may require supervision by a licensed healthcare practitioner, and thus they are not liable for any consequences from any recommendation, to any person reading or following the information in this book.

Table of Contents

Introduction

Many books have been written on shoulder pain.

This book is different.

It has been written to get right to the point.

To give you a clear understanding of the root causes of shoulder pain.

To give you a clear understanding of YOUR shoulder pain.

By the end of this book you should get 4 things:

1. A clear picture of what causes shoulder pain.

2. An understanding of the five MAIN causes of shoulder pain.

3. A clear picture of what is causing YOUR shoulder pain.

4. A plan of action to alleviate your shoulder pain.

The rest is up to you.

Enjoy the read

Best in health,

Chris

Chris Dukarski,PT

Let's Get Started

Shoulder pain is the third most common musculoskeletal disorder, following low back and neck pain

Did you realize that 75% of professional baseball pitchers have labral tears and 40% have rotator cuff tears but in most cases have no pain?

It certainly begs the question that a pitcher may need these tears in order to be able to throw a baseball close to 100 miles an hour.

Did you also realize that 60% of people over 60 years old have rotator cuff tears...yet no pain?

So why is it that some people with these tears experience pain yet others DO NOT?

If you have ever had shoulder pain, then you realize how dramatically your life can be affected.

Does it hurt when you reach overhead or get dressed?

Does it wake you up if you roll onto it?

Does it prevent you from throwing a ball to your child?

Yes, shoulder pain can be a real downer...unless you get the right treatment.

But first, you need to find out exactly WHAT to treat... before it's too late to fix it.

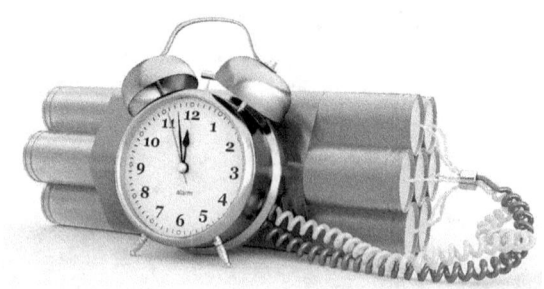

So then, WHAT exactly causes shoulder pain?

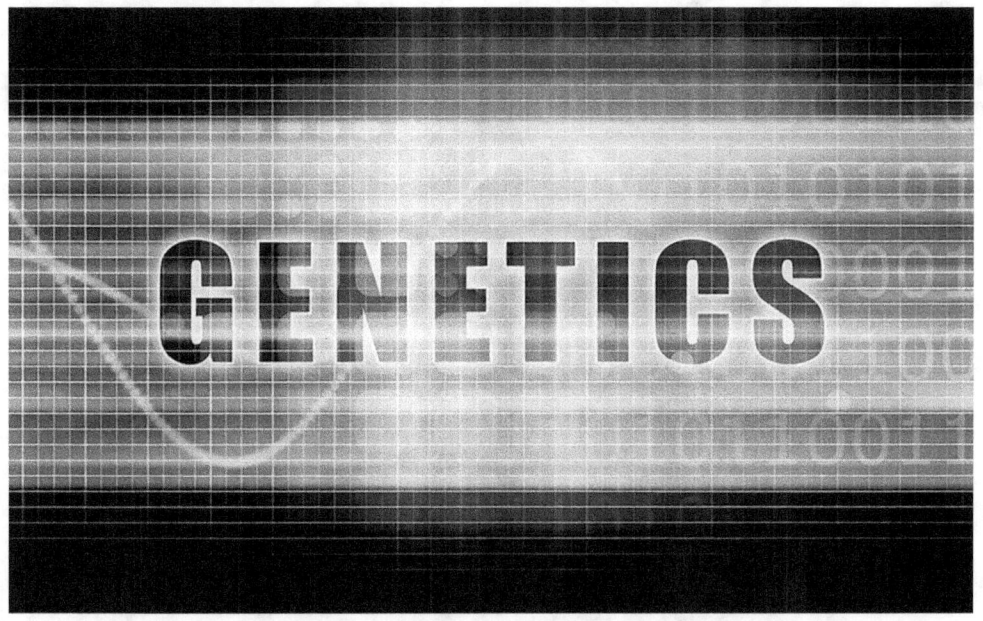

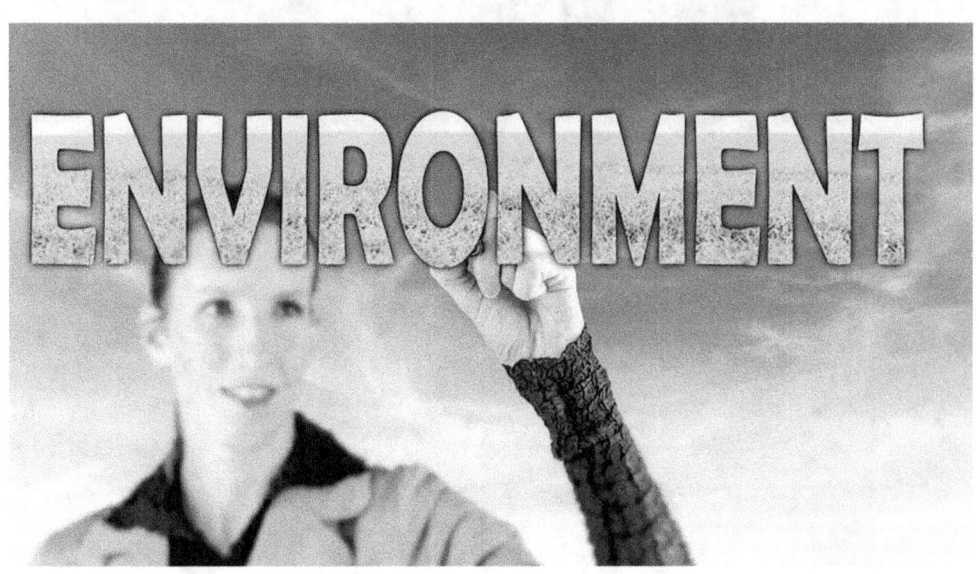

Genetically speaking, you are born with a specific code that you inherited from your parents.

How many times have you heard "Well, my mom (or dad) had a bad shoulder too."

You can't run away from your genes.

You just need to learn how to manage things better knowing that you have a family history of shoulder pain.

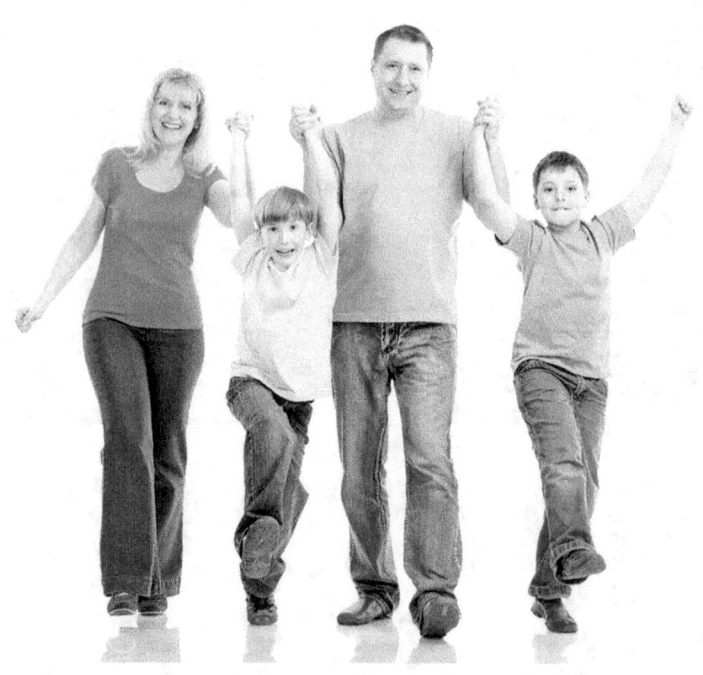

One of the biggest environmental influences:

The effects of GRAVITY!

As we age we become all too familiar with the effects of gravity.

As we stand upright, the effects of gravity on our bodies becomes much more significant.

Gravity has the effect of continuously pulling us down and, in most cases, pulling us forward thus causing us to slouch.

So how does slouching affect your shoulder?

Try this:

Slouch forward and really round out your back. Now try and raise your arm overhead. Feel the pinch?

Repeat this sitting straight up. Now try to raise your shoulder again. Much easier isn't it?

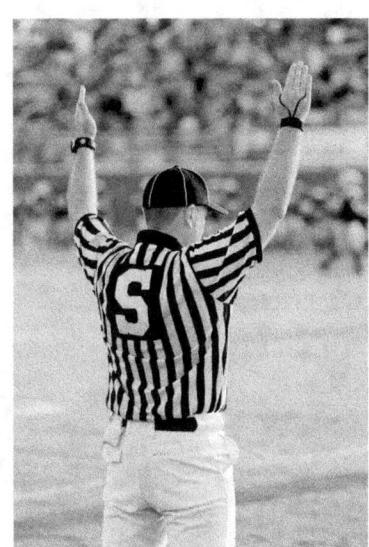

So what do your spinal curves have to do with it?

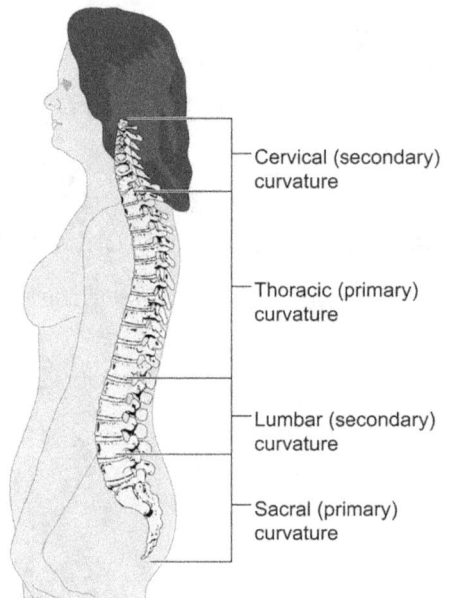

Cervical (secondary) curvature

Thoracic (primary) curvature

Lumbar (secondary) curvature

Sacral (primary) curvature

Structurally there are three distinct curves to a normal spine.

When the position of these three curves are maintained, you optimize your ability to function against gravity.

When they are not maintained, you set yourself up for injury to your shoulder.

So what exactly happens to the shoulder under these circumstances?

What most of us do not realize (until it's too late) is that these effects on the shoulder are cumulative.

The biggest question is not IF it will happen but….

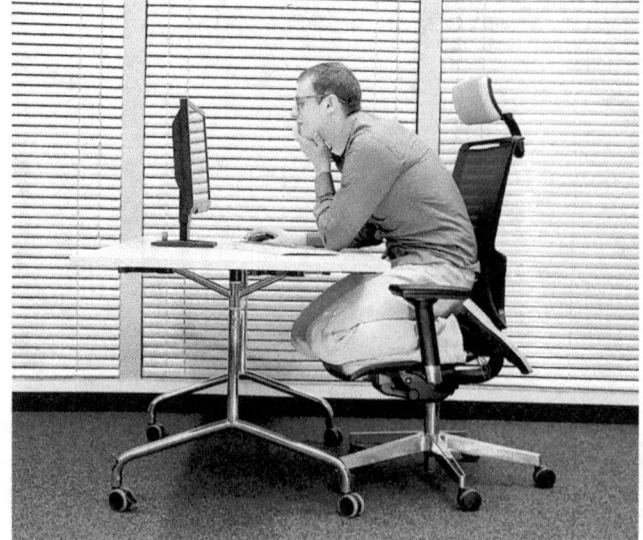

When it will happen?
&
How it will happen?

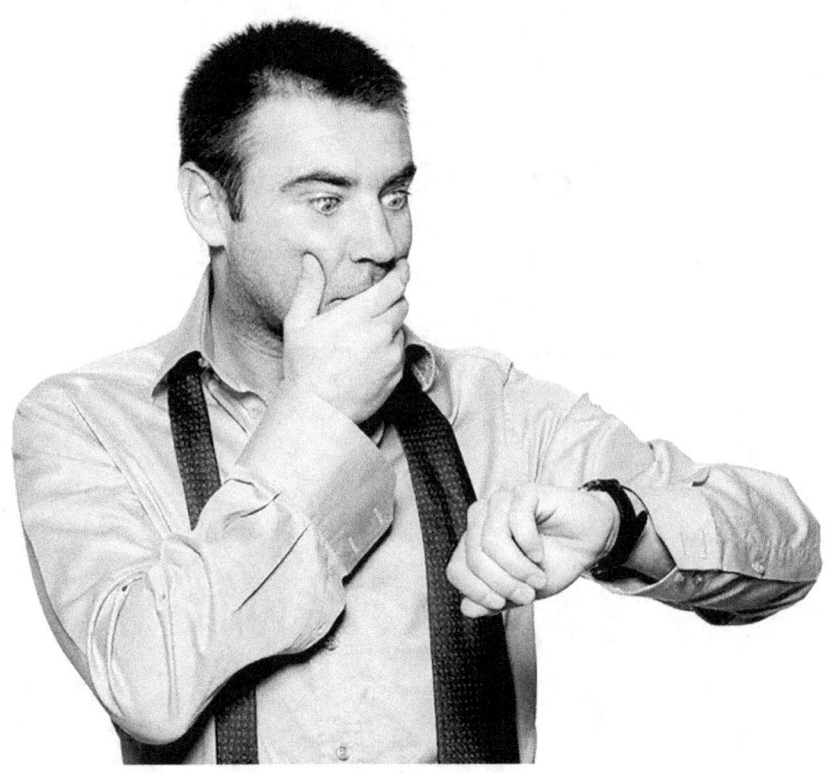

So what does your anatomy have to do with it?

Your shoulder joint is the most mobile joint in your body. It is formed by the articulation of the head of your humerus bone, your the shoulder blade or scapula and your collar bone or clavicle. There are 3 separate joints of the shoulder which you can see on the image below. The most problematic joint is the glenohumeral joint. This joint is a ball and socket joint and it is here where most of the motion in your shoulder occurs...and it is here where most of the problems arise.

Bones of the Shoulder

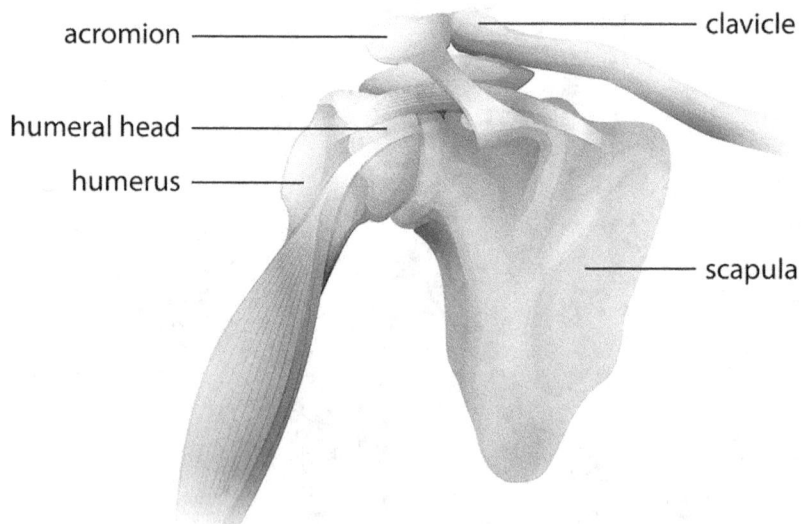

acromion ——————   —————— clavicle

humeral head ——————

humerus ——————

scapula

So what exactly happens to the shoulder under these conditions?

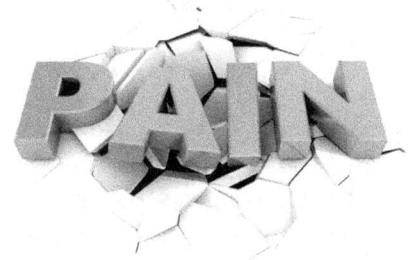

The five main causes of shoulder pain are:

- IMPINGEMENT SYNDROME or ROTATOR CUFF TENDONITIS

- ROTATOR CUFF OR LABRAL TEARS

- DEGENERATIVE CHANGES IN ONE OR SEVERAL OF THE 3 SHOULDER JOINTS

- SOFT TISSUE AND MUSCULAR IMBALANCES

- REFERRED PAIN FROM THE NECK

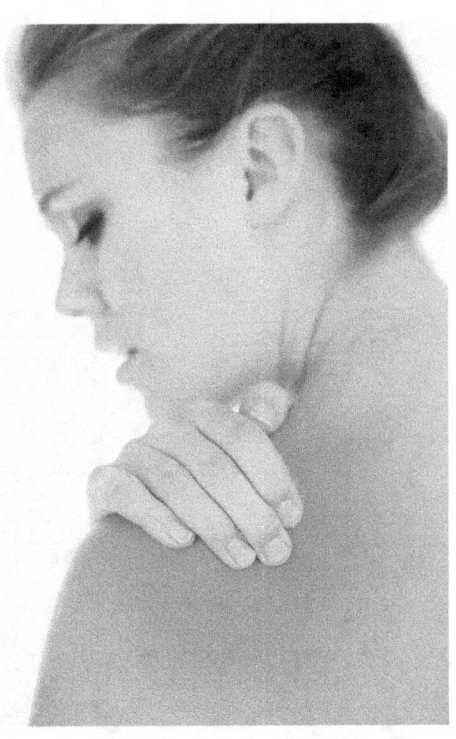

Problem #1: Shoulder Impingement Or Rotator Cuff Tendonitis

This is by far the most common cause of pain in the shoulder.

The main reason people experience an impingement or "pinching" in the shoulder is due to poor posture, poor body mechanics, and poor work ergonomics.

Just think about how many times you are slouched over your laptop or cell phone.

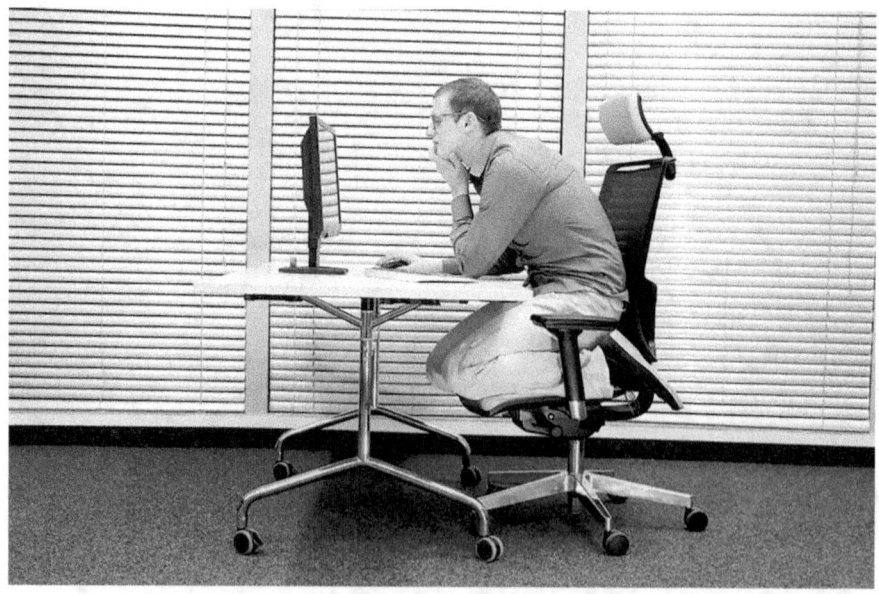

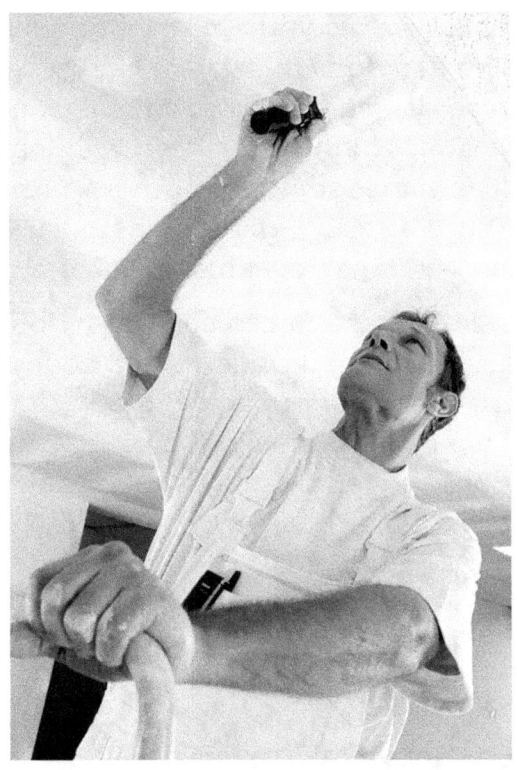

So what exactly IS impingement syndrome?

There is actually a certain amount of normal impingement in your shoulder. The soft tissue structures in the shoulder DO actually rub on the bony structures as you raise your arm but there is no pain in a healthy shoulder. So what rubs? Answer: your rotator cuff tendon!

Your rotator cuff tendon attaches to the top of your humerus and lies in between the humerus and the bottom part of the acromion process of your shoulder blade. This is called the sub-acromial space. With your arm hanging by your side, there should be a normal gap in the sub-acromial space. As you raise your arm this gap narrows.

Impingement results from a compromise in the sub-acromial space. Poor posture and body mechanics can mechanically narrow this space and cause damage to the soft tissue structures in the shoulder. This damage is further enhanced with the cumulative stresses of repetitive shoulder motion such as pitching or sustained overhead activity such as painting. This may initially lead to tendonitis or bursitis and then eventually to a rotator cuff tear.

Keep in mind that impingement can arise from both structural and functional causes. Yes, you could have a boney abnormality in the shoulder such as a spur or a malformed acromion process. But most often the pain from shoulder impingement arises from the stresses of poor posture, repetitive motion and soft tissue and muscular imbalances in the shoulder complex.

Normal   **Rotator cuff problems**

Inflamed/torn
tendons

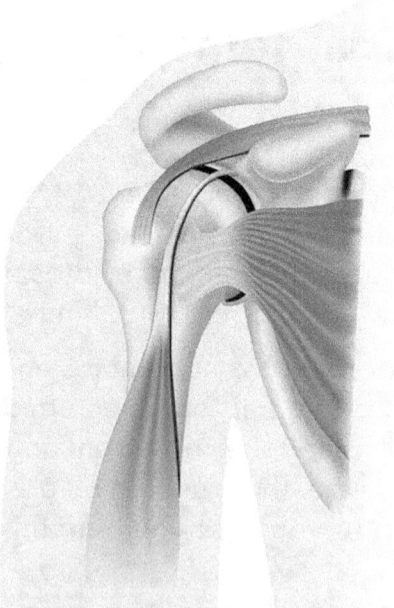
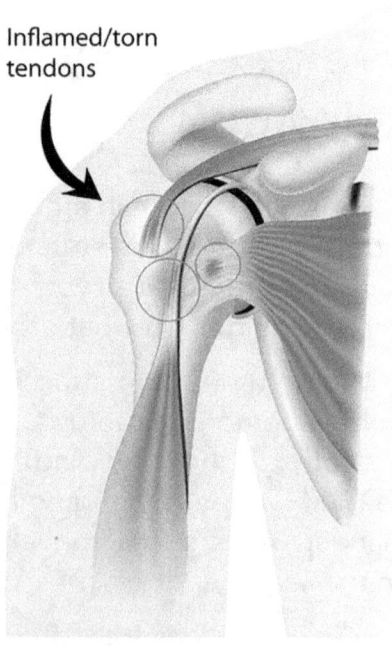

Problem #2: Rotator Cuff and Labral Tears

These are certainly the two most common tears that occur in the shoulder. As I mentioned earlier, 75% of professional pitchers have labral tears and 40% have rotator cuff tears. The prevalence of asymptomatic rotator cuff tears increases as we age and may be as high as 60% after 60 years old. So yes, you can have tears in these structures without experiencing any pain. Why you do or do not have pain is still unclear.

As mentioned earlier during our discussion on impingement syndrome, the rotator cuff can be damaged during repetitive stresses or direct trauma. This may eventually lead to a tear.

The labrum is a cartilage ring that deepens the fossa that holds the head of the humerus. It functions to provide extra stability to the glenohumeral joint. The labrum can be damaged through repetitive motion or direct trauma. This can lead to pain or instability of the shoulder.

The biggest take-home message from this is DO NOT rush off to surgery if an MRI confirms a labral or a rotator cuff tear. Many people can successfully rehab a shoulder with a tear and return to complete pain-free function WITHOUT surgery. It just takes time… and patience.

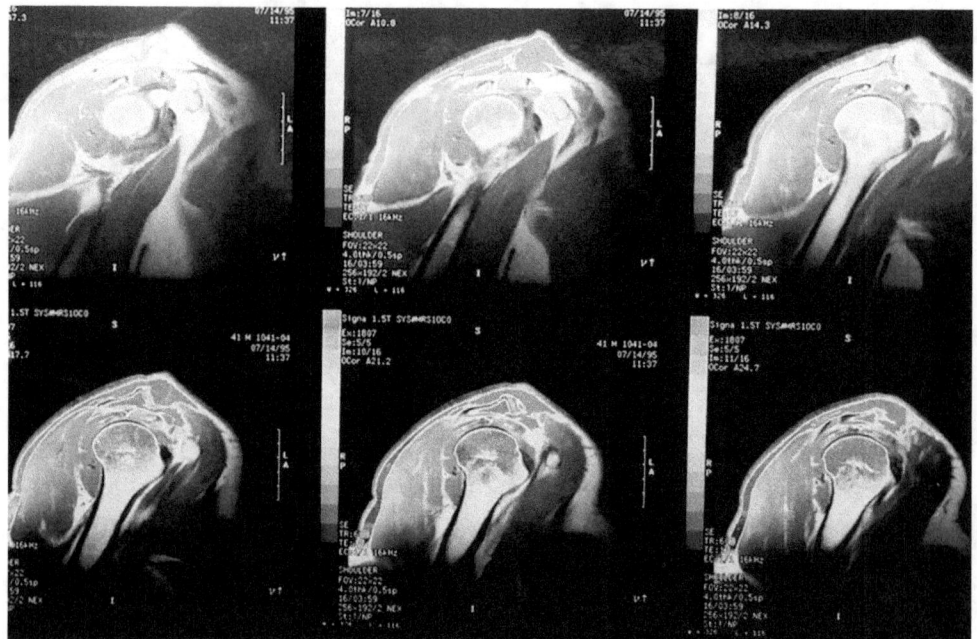

Problem #3: Degenerative Changes

The glenohumeral joint is the third most common large joint to be affected by arthritis. The first two being the knee and hip. The prevalence of shoulder arthritis in people over 60 years old is around 33%.

Wear and tear arthritis is called osteoarthritis. Because the shoulder joint is the most mobile joint in the human body, it is especially susceptible to wear and tear. Over time, the articular surfaces of the joints in the shoulder can wear out and bone can eventually rub on bone.

This degenerative process can occur in any one of the three joints in the shoulder complex. The 3 joints are the glenohumeral joint, the acromioclavicular joint, and the sternoclavicular joint.

Just because you have a diagnosis of arthritis, however, does not necessarily mean you will have pain.

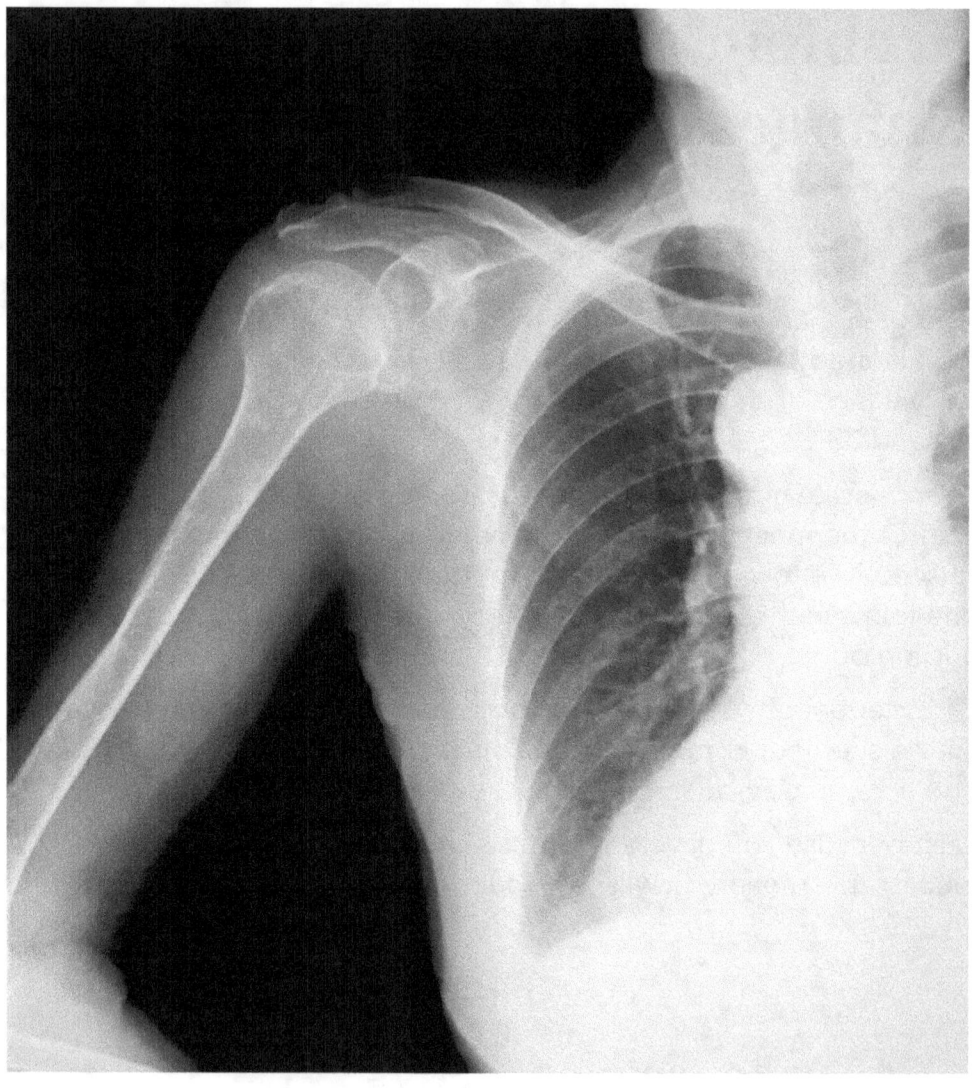

Problem #4: Soft Tissue and Muscle Imbalances

The most probable explanation for WHY people develop pain in the presence of degenerative tearing or arthritis in the shoulder is due to soft tissue and muscle imbalances. Pain develops when your normal movement patterns are altered. This occurs when you have insufficient strength, limited flexibility, or poor tissue quality.

Of course, as we age, we become weaker, stiffer, and our tissue quality deteriorates. There is an expected rhythm of motion between the three joints of your shoulder and an anticipated coordination of muscle contractions that occur to allow a full and pain-free elevation of your arm. If this is disrupted in anyway, it leads to imbalance. Unfortunately, most of us don't realize this imbalance is occurring until it's too late.

What's the first thing that people do when they experience a twinge of pain? Answer: compensations to AVOID the pain. This, of course, leads to further imbalance and continued deterioration of the joints in the shoulder. Chronic compensations can even lead to a frozen shoulder.

The best way to avoid these imbalances is to be proactive.

Consistency with a comprehensive program of strengthening, flexibility exercises, and soft tissue interventions is the key. The first step is a comprehensive bio-mechanical evaluation.

An ounce of prevention is worth a pound of cure!

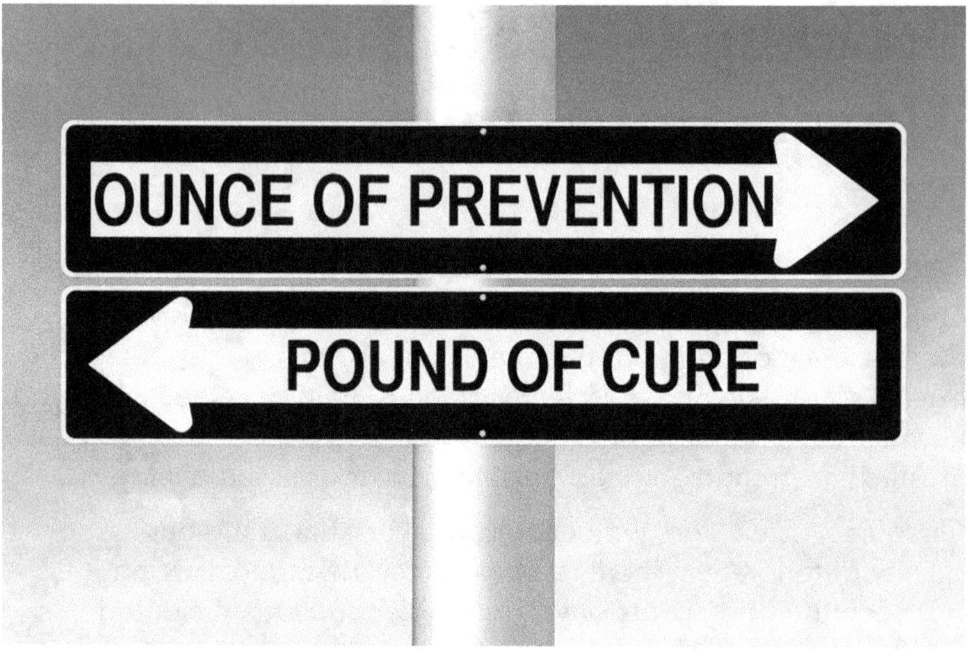
OUNCE OF PREVENTION
POUND OF CURE

Problem #5: Referred pain from the Neck

Have you ever heard of sciatica?

Sciatica results from a pinched nerve in your low back. In some circumstances, shoulder pain may be the result of a pinched nerve in your neck.

The more time that we spend slouched over our laptops and cell phones, the more opportunity there is for an impingement in your neck. This discussion is analogous to our discussion on shoulder impingement. The more that you compromise the available space for nerves or soft tissues to function, the more susceptible you are to having something pinched.

It is very important to determine whether your neck is contributing to your shoulder pain. As part of a comprehensive physical therapy evaluation, there are several tests that we use to determine this.

Do you still have shoulder pain even though you tried physical therapy?

Don't give up. There may be a good reason for that...

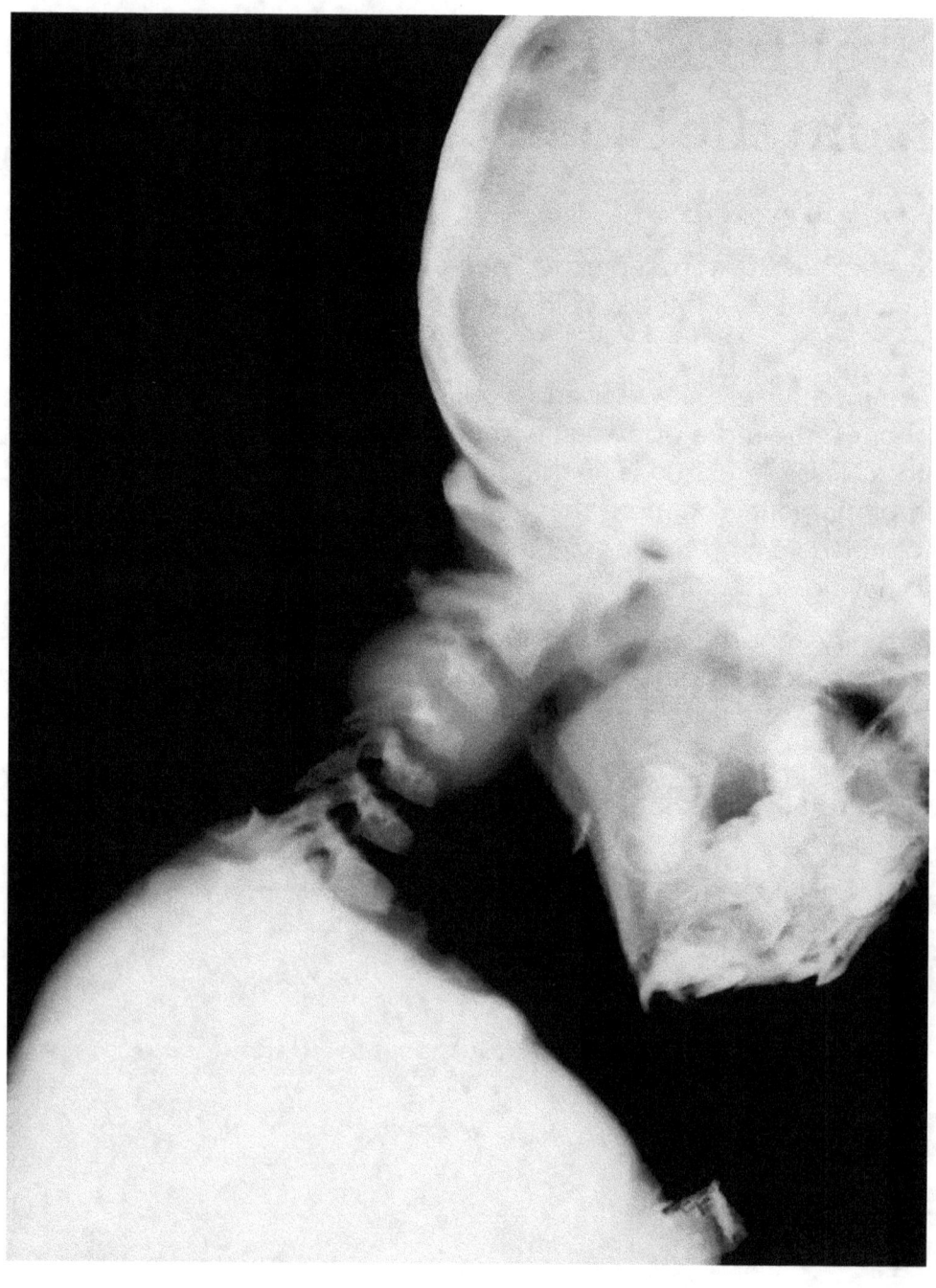

The next question is what do you do if you have shoulder pain?

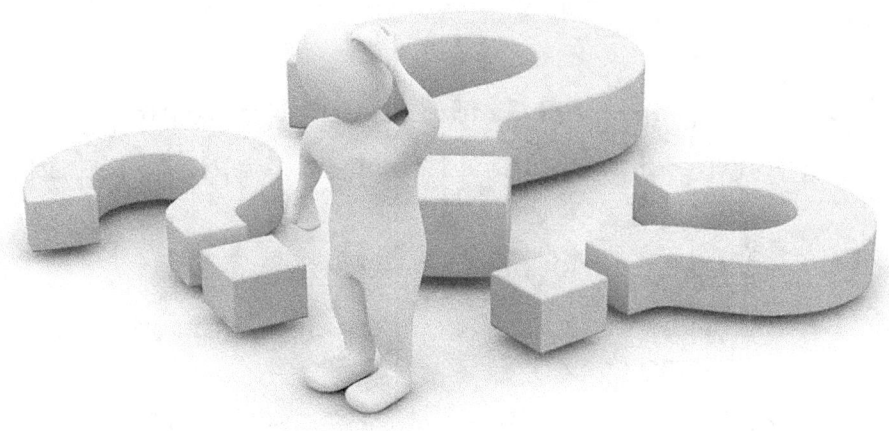

The Recipe for Success

So what is the first step to alleviating your pain?

The first step is to answer the necessary questions to determine exactly what the source of your pain is. There is a typical presentation to the 5 main causes of shoulder pain. As you will read, a "deep aching" is a common feature of several of the conditions. Lets begin.

#1: Shoulder Impingement Syndrome or RC tendonitis

1. Do you spend a lot of time slouched forward or hunched over your computer?

2. Do you perform a lot of overhead activity?

3. Do you have intermittent, point specific pain that occurs with overhead activity?

4. Do you have pain laying on your shoulder at night?

5. Can you reproduce your pain if you place your hand on the opposite shoulder and then raise your elbow up?

If you answered YES to these questions, then you could have a case of shoulder impingement syndrome or rotator cuff tendonitis.

#2a: Rotator Cuff Tear

1. Do you experience a deep aching in the shoulder?

2. Do you experience intermittent sharp pain with raising your arm overhead or reaching behind you?

3. Do you have pain when you lay on your arm?

4. Does your arm feel weak when you raise it?

5. Have you ever injured your shoulder with an episode of severe pain or tearing sensation?

If you answered YES to these questions, then you could have a rotator cuff tear.

#2b: Labral Tear

1. Do you experience popping, clicking, or catching in the shoulder.

2. Do you have pain when you move your arm over your head or throw a ball?

3. Do you have a feeling of weakness or instability in the shoulder?

4. Do you have a deep aching pain?

5. Do you have a hard time describing or pointing to exactly where the pain is?

6. Have you ever injured your shoulder with an episode of severe pain or tearing sensation?

If you answered YES to these questions, then you could have a labral tear.

#3: Degenerative arthritis of the shoulder

1. Do you experience a deep generalized aching of your shoulder?

2. Do you feel grinding or clicking in your shoulder as you raise it?

3. Do changes in weather affect your shoulder?

4. Do you have limited range of motion with dressing or reaching overhead question?

5. Does your arm feel weak or heavy?

If you answered YES to these questions, then you could have degenerative arthritis of the shoulder.

#4: Muscular and soft tissue imbalances

Most patients with shoulder pain will have some degree of muscular and soft tissue imbalances. The degree of the imbalance usually correlates with the chronicity of the problem.

#5: Referred Pain from Neck

1. Do you spend a lot of time slouching or hunched over your computer?

2. Do you have rounded shoulders?

3. Do you have concurrent neck and upper back stiffness or soreness?

4. Do you experience shoulder pain when you move your neck?

5. Do you experience any numbness or tingling in your shoulder or arm?

If you answered YES to these questions, then you could have referred pain into your shoulder from your neck

Best Treatment Strategy

EDUCATION

Knowledge is Power!

You're first step in recovery is understanding your condition and understanding the best way to treat it.

The second step is realizing that if your shoulder pain is reproducible, it is probably reducible.

So lets give you a plan of action to reduce it and alleviate it once and for all.

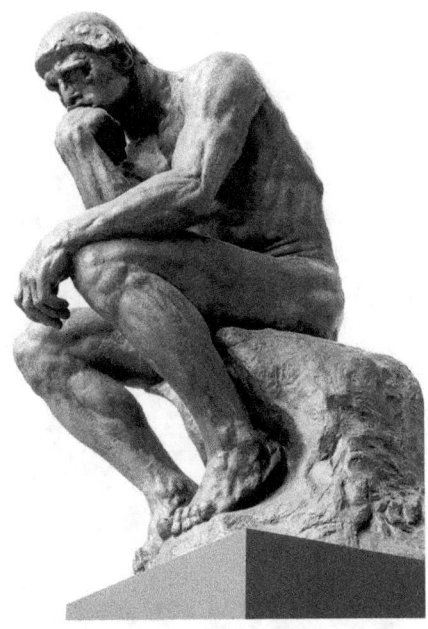

Step #1:

Go to my You Tube channel at http://bit.ly/Best3Strategies to get started.

My videos will explain the Best 3 Strategies to treat shoulder pain.

The content of these videos is applicable to ANY of the aforementioned causes of shoulder pain.

You need to create a foundation to heal and these videos will provide that.

Step #2:

Go to my You Tube channel at http://bit.ly/Best3Strategies to continue.

The Best Exercises for shoulder pain will be presented in each of the videos on my Best Exercises playlist.

In Conclusion

Low back pain is a treatable and curable condition.

Can you change your genetics? NO. But you can manage the influence of the environment upon it.

The first step is understanding your condition.

The second step is following a recipe for success with an effective plan of action.

The third is looking for a qualified physical therapist if you are not successful in resolving your pain with steps 1 and 2.

Give me a call at OrthoWell Physical Therapy if you need my help.

Beverly, MA 978-522-4199

Newburyport,MA 978-462-2700

info@orthowellpt.com

Best in Health,

Chris Dukarski,PT

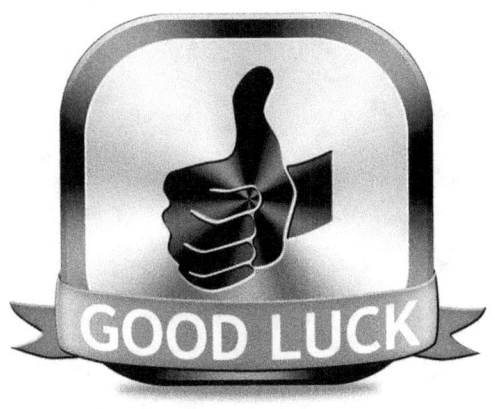